Electronic Cigarette:

The Beginners Guide To e-Cigarettes, Vaping & E-Hookah

by Victor Fields

Table of Contents

Copyright

Under no circumstances will any legal responsibility or blame be held against the publisher for any reparation, damages, or monetary loss due to the information herein, either directly or indirectly.

Respective authors own all copyrights not held by the publisher.

The information herein is offered for informational purposes solely, and is universal as so. The presentation of the information is without contract or any type of guarantee assurance.

The trademarks that are used are without any consent, and the publication of the trademark is without permission or backing by the trademark owner. All trademarks and brands within this book are for clarifying purposes only and are the owned by the owners themselves, not affiliated with this document.

Introduction

It's a given fact: Smoking is a nasty habit. There are so many diseases attributed to smoking that listing everything down would need a chapter dedicated to it. If there's one disease that is readily associated with smoking, it is lung cancer.

But how can we as a nation eradicate this vice? With over 40 million smokers in the states alone, eradicating smoking is going to create a massive upheaval in the economic infrastructure.

Although it's not something a lot of people would understand as a good thing, tobacco companies employ a lot of people to work in their tobacco fields and cigarette manufacturing plants. Taking out smoking is going to affect the lives of all these people and it may take years for them to recover if they ever do at all.

Stricter laws have been put in place and they do seem to work in curbing this type of addiction but it does not solve the problem entirely. In fact, a direct result of these laws is a higher tax levied against tobacco smokers. And we all know that you can only jack the price up so much before these people start rising up and lobbying for fairer rules and regulations.

So what can we do to appease the people who still want to smoke and make sure that it is safer than regular tobacco smoke?

It seems like technology has once again provided us with a solution to our everyday problem and come up with an ingenious way to provide smokers with the ability to smoke without endangering a lot of people around them.

Based on an ancient Persian technology called the Hookah, these e-cigarettes seem to be popping up everywhere and it is becoming readily available to people all around the world. It has also helped lots of people who are heavily addicted to smoking to transition from a costly habit to a safer alternative.

Today, the term "Vaping" has become popular. With a lot of enthusiasts choosing to take the safer route, the e-cigarette market has seen a rise in popularity and their market share has become considerably huge.

This book will give you an idea about the pros and cons involving e-cigarettes, vaping and e-hookahs.

Chapter 1. What Is An E-Cigarette?

Electronic cigarettes or e-Cigarettes as they've become known for are basically gadgets designed to look and feel like real cigarettes and provide the sensation of smoking to smokers all over the world without the harmful effects of real tobacco cigarettes.

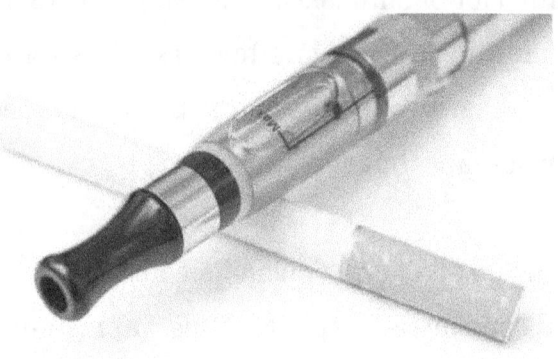

The basic operation for these devices involve the use of essential oils in a fabric heated to emanate smoke from.

There is no burning involved.

Now some e-Cigarettes may look so realistic and even have the "lighted tip" light up as bright as real cigarettes but this is just an illusion to help the smoker's mind accept the fact that they are in fact "smoking".

E-Cigarettes came into existence thanks to ancient Persian technology and surprisingly some medical devices. The e-Cigarette is in actuality a vaporizer. Hence the term "vaping" when you're using an e-Cigarette.

E-Cigarettes first came into the public's eye around the early part of 2008. The first versions were made to look exactly like real cigarettes and these were produced in China. Early reception of these devices was basically lukewarm and people tended to pass it off as a novelty item.

But long time cigarette smokers who wanted to quit smoking saw it as a device that could help them get off real tobacco cigarettes and choose e-Cigarettes as a safer alternative. It didn't take long for these items to become more popular and with the help of aggressive promotions as well as improvements; these gadgets have become common place.

Nowadays, e-Cigarettes are no longer treated as a novelty item. It has in fact spawned pockets of enthusiasts all over the world who swear by the usage of these items as very helpful to their recovery from tobacco.

Now, how does an e-Cigarette work?
As mentioned before, e-Cigarettes are basically vaporizers. There is no actual smoke coming out of it. It is instead an aerosol which is mostly water that comes out from the mouths of the "vapers" (people who use e-Cigarettes).

The basic construction of an e-Cigarette mostly comes in a cylindrical form (to better emulate the shape of a cigarette) and is no bigger than an actual stick of tobacco. It is also painted to look the same way. But that is basically where the resemblance ends.

Since e-Cigarettes use a battery and an atomizer, there is a considerable weight difference. Whereas a stick of real tobacco cigarette may only weigh a couple of grams, an e-cigarette can weigh more than two packs of cigarettes. That's not a huge weight difference but it does exist. An e-Cigarette is also comprised of plastic or metal parts which basically feel different when compared with real cigarettes which are wrapped in paper instead. And last but not the least, since e-Cigarettes are more solidly constructed, there is that lack of give when you place the device in your mouth or hold it between your fingers.

Chapter 2. E-Cigarettes, Basic Parts

This self-contained device does not need an external flame source to light it up. As long as the batteries are charged, it will provide the necessary energy to allow the Atomizer to heat up the fabric which is doused with the e-Liquid.

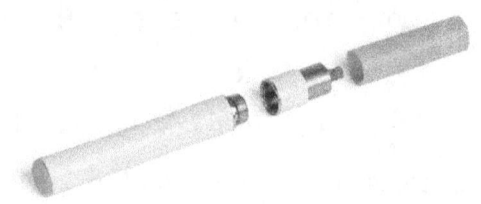

(image from: blog.my7s.com)

1. Mouthpiece
2. Atomizer
3. Battery
4. LED light

These 4 are constructed so well that at first

glance you would be convinced that you have a real stick of tobacco in front of you until you pick it up.

1. **Mouthpiece**

   The mouthpiece or the cartridge is usually where the e-Liquid is housed in. This is the part that touches our mouths. It is often porous in design in order to allow vapor to seep through from the device to our mouths.

2. **Atomizer**

   Perhaps the atomizer is the most important part of the e-Cigarette, but then that's still up for debate. This is where the magic happens. The atomizer is the one responsible for heating up the e-Liquid and turning it into an aerosol which when released into the air looks like thick smoke.

3. **Battery**

   Of course, since the e-Cigarette is an

electronic gadget, it would need something to power it. Small lithium ion batteries are used for e-Hookahs while e-Cigarettes are relegated to using the batteries normally found in watches.

4. **LED light**

Perhaps the only important part that serves only as an aesthetic purpose.

The LED light is usually placed at the tip of the e-Cigarette where it is supposed to be "burning". Like a real tobacco cigarette, these LED lights are programmed to increase their luminescence the stronger you inhale.

The manner in which these e-Cigarettes are used is often through this method:

1. Turn on the device

2. Bring the e-Cigarette's mouthpiece to your mouth and start inhaling as if it were a real stick of tobacco cigarette.

3. The device's atomizer then heats up the e-Liquid to produce an aerosol that is released through the air like a real cigarette smoke.

4. As soon as you've had your fill of smoke in your mouth and lungs, remove the e-Cigarette from your mouth and exhale.

The process is instantaneous and provides an experience like smoking a real cigarette. This is basically the same for the e-Hookah as well.

Chapter 3: Guide to Hookahs

Like mentioned, in the previous chapter, using an -ehookah is the almost the same as vaping. When you buy your first e-Cigarette or e-Hookah it would be best to do it in the actual shop so you can test out the product and make sure that it is the right fit for you.

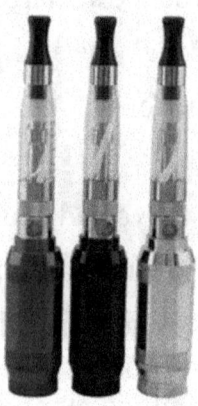

(image from: www.arabamericannews.com)

You can also have modifications done to it if you want it to burn faster or slower just by having the coils adjusted.

You'll also have access to the many different e-Liquids available in most shops. They can let you test it out for yourself by applying a few drops and letting you taste the e-Liquid.

If you are going to do this, make sure you don't overdo it. Inhale just a few breaths of the e-Liquid, swirl it around your mouth and exhale. This should give you a basic idea of what you're getting.

For e-Hookahs, there are two types that you can buy.

The first one which is the most commonly sold one is the pen type e-Hookah. It is slightly larger than an e-Cigarette and doesn't look anything at all like a real cigarette. It is often just a cylindrical metal shape with the necessary components in it like the mouthpiece, the atomizer and the battery units. These gadgets also last longer than the usual e-Cigarette since they utilize bigger batteries.

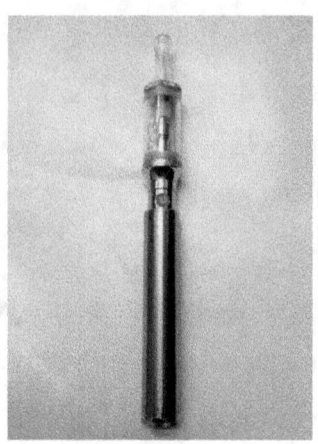

(image from: cmbvapors.com)

The smoke you can derive from e-Hookahs are also considerably heavier since the atomizers are more efficient in heating up the coil soaked in the e-Liquid.

Nowadays it seems like more and more people are using the e-Hookah instead of the e-Cigarette.

The other type of e-Hookah is the one with many mouthpieces attached to it.

It looks just like the traditional Persian hookah and is fun for social events.

The basic usage is just the same except this time 2 or more people (usually 4) can partake with one single inhalation.

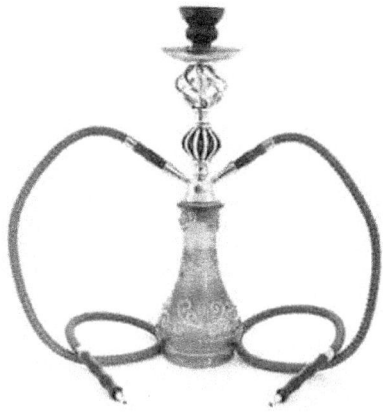

(image from: www.shishaa.co.uk)

These e-hookahs are especially fun during social events and are great conversation starters.

Chapter 4: E-Liquids

Now let's talk about e-Liquids. Without e-Liquids, you won't be able to produce the aerosol which is the "smoke" you derive from these e-Cigarettes and e-Hookahs.

E-Liquids come in little bottles and are easily administered into the coil inside your device. You will have to unscrew the top of your e-Cigarette or e-Hookah to place the liquid on the coil though. It's a very simple operation and it usually just takes a couple of seconds to do it. Before you know it, you've got your e-Cigarette top screwed back on and you can start puffing away.

The fun thing about e-Liquids which maybe is one of the main selling points of e-Cigarettes is that they provide vapers with different flavors. The normal e-Liquid you'd find is the nicotine flavored one.

But, if you're the adventurous type, you can experiment with e-Liquids that are strawberry flavored, watermelon flavored and other fruity flavors. Once you inhale the aerosol into your mouth you'll be able to taste a hint of the fruity flavor you chose and when you exhale it, the scent is basically the same!

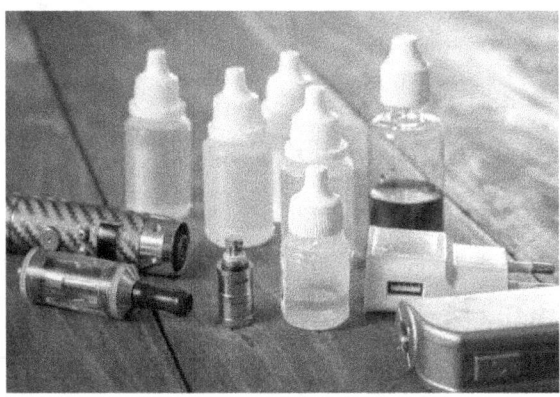

Chapter 5. Making the Switch to E-Cigs

There are over 40 million smokers in the US alone. That's a lot of smokers to contend with. And there are a lot of tobacco companies willing to serve these smokers any particular brand they want. And if it hasn't been repeated enough times already: Smoking is dangerous to your health.

So what makes smoking so dangerous and why do people still do it?

Well, first off, why do people do it: You'll have to thank the many advertising companies who have succeeded in imbedding the image that smoking is cool!

You see it everywhere you go, from print ads to video ads. Everyone who wants to be regarded as cool is seen with a cigarette in their mouth.

One of the most iconic images in the world is that of the Marlboro man. This man has all the qualities needed to convince any man out there that in order to be a man, they'd need to dress like him, move like him and even smoke like him. But that's just the power of advertising.

What makes smoking addicting is the nicotine additive, giving the user a feeling of pleasure. It is what makes it quite difficult to quit smoking. No one really looks into the fine print involved in cigarettes. There are too many lung damage cases in the world attributed to smoking cigarettes as well as to second hand smoke. If we must list down all of the diseases that smoking contributes to, it'd require a whole other chapter. But for the curious, smoking affects each and every part of our body from our eyes to our liver and most definitely our lungs.

It has been the leading cause of cancer and it saps our bodies of energy we need to function because our cardiovascular system is compromised.

Aside from the damage it does to our bodies, smoking is also bad for the environment.
And have you ever wondered what happened to the Marlboro man? Well he did get to live to a ripe old age of 85, but it wasn't without the presence of lung damage. He also lobbied against cigarette smoking and raised awareness for young people not to take up the habit of smoking even though it did look cool!

Chapter 6. Benefits of vaping

"If you must take a risk, at least choose the less deadly one."

This seems to be the idea behind vaping.

Although e-Cigarettes are regarded as a better alternative to actual smoking it does come with its own dangers.

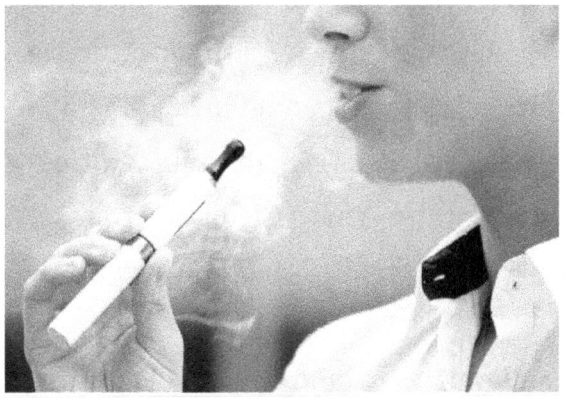

(image from: http://www.nypost.com)

Now, the reason why vaping seems to be popular nowadays is because of the fact that smokers who want to lessen their evil habits but still want to retain the sense of smoking have chosen to live in this manner.

There are many ways to stop smoking. There are also many products out there that can help you decrease your dependency to cigarettes but there is absolutely no product yet out there that emulates smoking with lesser harm to one's own body than that of e-Cigarettes.

With vaping, you are inhaling fewer chemicals than the ones you'd find in a stick of cigarette. The active components found in an e-Liquid are: propylene glycol, vegetable oil, flavoring and distilled water. This is significantly less than what you'd find in a cigarette stick.

Vaping allows you to enjoy the act of smoking (bringing your hand to your mouth and inhaling smoke from the cigarette) without the use of tobacco products and tricks your mind to believing that you are still smoking the real stuff.

This helps long time smokers slowly wean themselves off of tobacco cigarettes and hasten their path to recovery from smoking addiction. Another benefit that you can derive from vaping is that: since it is basically an aerosol, there are lesser pollutants released into the air around you.

After using your e-Cigarette or e-Hookah, you don't need to throw it away. You can just as easily stow it back into its carrying case until the next time you want to take a few puffs. That means no more cigarette butts on the ground. There's also no ash involved when smoking your e-Cigarette. Since it is a self-contained device, there is no ash present which can bring about allergies as well as dirty up your place.

e-Cigarettes or e-Hookahs are rechargeable so there is no need to continue buying a new device every time you've ran out of batteries.

Just pop it into any available socket and wait for it to fully charge before you use it again.

And last but not the least, there are so many e-Liquid flavors out there that you can experiment with. You can have the plain old nicotine taste or you can choose to get a strawberry flavored and scented e-Liquid. This is one of the main selling points of e-Cigarettes. The ability to choose flavors is particularly enticing to long time smokers who want to experiment with something new.

Chapter 7. The pros and cons of e-cigarettes

So are e-Cigarettes really all that healthy? Well, yes and no. Although there are considerably less health hazards involved with e-Cigarettes, take note that they have yet to be approved by the FDA as a truly healthy alternative to tobacco smoking.

We'll let you find out and decide for your own self.

We've listed down as many pros and cons involving e-Cigarettes and let you choose if you want to take up the habit of vaping instead of smoking.

Pros

1. No actual burning takes place
One of the things that truly peeves people off whether they are smokers or not is the presence of ash after lighting up a cigarette.

If you've ever been in a place where smokers usually converge in, you'll not only see a lot of cigarette butts but also the presence of too much ash which can be quite irritating!

This is one of the main selling points e-Cigarettes have. Since it is a self-contained unit and it relies on heating up a fabric to activate the e-Liquid, there is no real burning that actually happens.

2. You can throw your lighters away
Another issue that e-Cigarettes seem to have solved is the "Lost Lighter syndrome". Smokers tend to misplace lighters or hand it to someone who doesn't give it back.

With e-Cigarettes, you won't have to worry about that since the device heats up the coil inside its body to produce vapors.

So now you can do away with all of those lighters and have a self-contained smoking device ready for you to use at any time you want without having to search for a lighter.

3. It lets you wean off nicotine.
Nicotine is still present in e-Cigarettes. Most e-Liquids have a dose of nicotine in them to emulate the taste of real tobacco.
But the good news is you can wean yourself off nicotine and overcome your condition if you use e-liquids with small amounts of nicotine. Do not do anything drastic – it should be gradual. Reduce the nicotine amounts over time and you'll be fine.

4. The FDA is working towards regulating e-Cigarettes in the near future
As with any product that's out there today, the FDA is making the right move to regulate e-Cigarettes and e-Hookahs.

Since using these gadgets mean you would be taking substances into your body via the vapors, it is a concern related to your health.

Although most manufacturers would say that these products are only meant for recreational purposes, it is in our best interest for these to be properly regulated by the FDA to ensure that any health risks we face can be reduced in the near future.

There are also companies that produce these gadgets without any form of quality control on site which resulted in inferior products which do not work according to how it should.

And lastly, there are also companies that produce these gadgets without any form of quality control on site which resulted in inferior products which do not work according to how it should.

5.   E-Cigarettes can save you some money in the long run

Cigarette smokers all over the world know just how costly a smoking habit can be.
One stick of tobacco cigarettes can last for a minute or two depending on the number of puffs one smoker takes as well as the conditions of the environment. That means, if you chain smoke, one pack of cigarettes will only last you for about an hour or an hour and a half tops if you take a small break between cigarettes.

e-Cigarettes on the other hand can last for as long as your batteries can hold out and you can take as many puffs as you want without having to dispose of it.

So in effect, an e-Cigarette is worth more than a couple of packs of tobacco cigarettes which makes it a very good purchase for its ability to save you some money.

The only thing you would need to keep on purchasing would be the e-Liquid which you have to restock in your cartridge every so often.

6. You can vape anywhere you want to

Since vaping basically produces vapors and not smoke, many establishments have allowed the use of e-Cigarettes and e-Hookahs within their premises.

That means you won't have to walk a considerable distance just so you can partake in your favorite past time which is producing "smoke". It is still possible to inhale second hand vapor.

Just because vaping doesn't really produce smoke doesn't mean you can just vape in a crowd. It is still considered extremely rude to blow vapors into someone's face.

So if you do want to vape, at least vape away from other people. It is possible for them to inhale second hand vapor, although it would not be as harmful as cigarette smoke. Be considerate, other people will thank you for it.

Cons

1.   There's little to none in terms of Quality Control... yet.
2.   As a fairly new product that is offered openly to the market, e-Cigarettes have yet to go through stringent quality control management.

As such there are unscrupulous companies that have been offering sub-par products which may cause injuries to the user or not work according to how it should. There are also e-Liquids which are dubious in how it was created which may also prove hazardous to the users' health.

3. e-Cigarettes have been known to combust if

you do not know how to use them

4.   This is usually attributed to user error. Usually, e-Cigarettes are charged up to the point where the small batteries can no longer contain the power surging through them causing it to explode. Although we use explode as the term here, it usually just means that the batteries made a small pop and need to be replaced.

There are also instances wherein the e-Cigarettes are subjected to too much moisture. It could be because they were exposed to open air for an extended period of time or the humidity in our pockets caused moisture to penetrate the device.

There are also people who made modifications to their e-Cigarettes or e-Hookahs which resulted in an incompatibility in the parts leading to a malfunction.

Whatever the case, e-Cigarettes should be handled with care especially since we operate it too near to our face. To reduce the risk of this happening to you, make sure you purchase one from a reliable source who also has technical staff to support you when the need arises.

Let's face it: an e-Cigarette doesn't feel exactly like a cigarette, doesn't look exactly like one and it doesn't even weigh exactly like one. What it does is emulate cigarette smoking which nicotine pads or gum can never reproduce.

It allows you to continue on with the habit of bringing a cigarette into your mouth, inhaling the smoke and then releasing it into the air before bringing your hand back down. This is a cycle most smokers readily identify with.

It can help wean you off of excessive smoking though.

Chapter 8. Vaping lifestyle

So now that you have this information with you about e-cigarettes, e-hookahs and vaping, it is now entirely up to you to make that choice whether to continue smoking regular tobacco brands or to do away with all of that and choose a safer alternative to smoking.

Please understand that although vaping is considered as a safer alternative to actually inhaling smoke derived from tobacco, it does come with a few health hazards.

Choosing to smoke e-cigarettes not only will improve your health but can also save you a couple hundred dollars. If you think about it, smoking a pack a day can run up a total annual spending on cigarettes alone at a minimum of a thousand dollars a year.

That number does not include the amount of money you will be spending on disposable lighters, lighter fluid or matches.

And then there's the hassle of trying to find a place to smoke which can mean a lot of walking just so the local authorities won't fine you for smoking in unregulated places.

So you see, tobacco smoking may be deemed cool to the public eye but that doesn't mean it doesn't come with a few hassles along the way. If these TV ads and other promotional materials ever showed that, people probably won't be smoking that much.

Whereas, buying an e-cigarette will only cost you around a hundred bucks depending on the type of e-cigarette you want to get. You can make modifications which you can do by yourself or with the help of a local vape shop who specializes in it.

This will cost you a few dollars more and the essential oils needed for vaping purposes cost anywhere from five to 10 dollars depending on the store you bought it from.

There are also many types of scents that you can choose from which can range from the basic nicotine flavored vaping solution to others that are more exotic and aromatic like jasmine and myrrh.

So how do I go about becoming part of the vaping lifestyle?

Basically, just buying an e-Cigarette or an e-Hookah will immediately make you a part of the vaping lifestyle.

Make sure you buy from a trusted source of e-Cigarettes and e-Hookahs as well as e-Liquid.

Although the e-Cigarette industry is still unregulated, that doesn't mean there aren't any companies out there working towards improving the current technology involved in making these vaporizers. They are now safer than ever before and the e-Liquid that comes along with it have also been developed to have lesser harsh chemicals in it than what was previously offered. Hopefully, tobacco companies all over the world can find a way to adjust to this new change in lifestyle and come up with products that focus on providing healthier options to smokers not just in the states but in other countries as well.

We do have to remember that these companies also provide jobs to people and losing their employment can wreak havoc on their lives. Who knows, maybe these companies can come up with safer e-cigarettes and e-hookahs with the oils to match!

Conclusion

Now that you have all this, it is entirely up to you if you still want to continue with your decision to take up vaping or not.

What we've done is lay down the facts so that you know what you're getting into and not regret that you were misinformed.

The good thing is that the e-Cigarette market is still growing and these devices are getting more improvements every day to make them safer for the regular consumer. So always check back for more information about e-Cigarettes so you'll know what you're getting yourself into.

As an addiction, it is understandable that smoking can be hard to remove from one's life but with the help of modern technology, you now have an option to slowly wean yourself off of tobacco smoking and finally have a healthier lifestyle. Aside from e-cigarettes, you do have the option to quit smoking through the use of nicotine patches, nicotine gums, hypnotherapy or meditation. It all depends on your willingness to take that step to saying goodbye to the bad habit permanently.

In conclusion, vaping may be considered a fad today but it is quickly gaining enough market share that tobacco companies have started looking into developing e-Liquids as well as safer and better e-Cigarettes to consumers all over the world!

In the end, the choice is entirely yours to make.